Your Amazing
Itty Bitty™
Marijuana Manual

15 Ways to Use Cannabis for Your Health

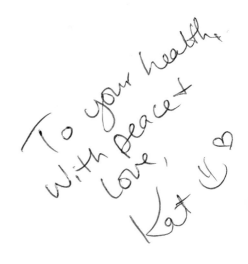

To your healthy
with peace +
love,
Kat 💛

Kat Bohnsack

Published by Itty Bitty™ Publishing
A subsidiary of S & P Productions, Inc.

Printed in the United States of America

Itty Bitty™ Publishing
311 Main Street, Suite E
El Segundo, CA 90245
(310) 640-8885

ISBN: 978-1-931191-75-3

This book is dedicated to Vivian McPeak and all of the people on this planet who use cannabis (marijuana) (as it has been used for thousands of years) for their health and believe in the amazing healing powers of this incredible medicinal plant. May we continue to educate, heal and use what God gave us for the greater good of this planet. And to my parents who on SO MANY levels, this book would not have been possible without. I love you to the moon and back!

To get your **FREE GIFT** – the groundbreaking creative visualization – "Money-Mind Mastery: Make More Money With The Power Of Your Mind"– **Text** 55678. **Enter the code**: "ITTY BITTY," in message box and enjoy.

Table of Contents

Introduction

This book is designed to be used solely for informational purposes. It is the result of years of research designed to bring you the most accurate information possible with regards to holistic cannabis practices that are being used to treat a variety of conditions today.

Cannabis has been used for thousands of years in many cultures for many reasons. There are terms in this book that will be used frequently, and to aid in comprehending the given information, the abbreviated definitions are given here.

Cannabis – The Cannabis Sativa L., a flowering hemp (marijuana) plant used for medicinal purposes for thousands of years. The two most common subspecies are Indica and Sativa; also referred to in this book as marijuana, pot or medicine.

Cannabinoids – The active compounds from the cannabis plant that are widely acclaimed for their healing properties.

CBD's – Cannabinoids, specifically Cannabidiol.

THC - Tetrahydrocannabinol, the chemical responsible for most of marijuana's psychological effects. It is resin from the cannabis plant and it shows up as clear or milky white "crystals" on the flower buds, leaves and stem.

Edible – Any food or drink that is made with some form of cannabis and therefore is "medicated" to give you a chosen effect.

Topical – A medicinal lotion, cream or oil applied directly to the skin for restorative effects. Topicals will not "get you high" or should not have any psychoactive effects.

Vaping – A way to safely inhale dried leaf cannabis or cannabis oil without smoke entering the lungs. The heating element heats the THC "crystals" and melts them, turning them into vapor, which is inhaled.

Indica – A subspecies of cannabis that provides a strong body high, relaxation, sedative and calming effect.

Sativa – A subspecies of cannabis that provides a head high that can include uplifting feeling, euphoria.

Hybrid – A combination of an Indica and Sativa strain giving the user both benefits of the "cross-strain."

Health Tips

Health Tip 1
Cannabis vs. Cancer

For many years the debate has rolled on about whether smoking or ingesting pot can help someone with cancer.

1. *"Cannabis* has been used for medicinal purposes for thousands of years." – Cancer.gov
2. "Over twenty major studies in the past nine years have shown that cannabinoids (the chemicals in cannabis) actually fight cancer cells." – Medicalmarijuana.com
3. Vaping (smoking cannabis leaf in vapor form), smoking or eating edibles have all shown to be effective in helping some people with different types of cancers get relief from pain, retain their hair during chemo, soothe nausea, encourage appetite, heal faster and have clean bills of health from cancer, as well as other ailments.
4. "Over the past few years, research has revealed that marijuana can both destroy certain cancer cells and reduce the growth of others." – Huffingtonpost.com

Cannabis vs. Cancer

- Cancers where marijuana treatment has shown effectiveness include:
  - Brain tumors/cancer
  - Lung cancer
  - Breast cancer
  - Leukemia
  - Melanoma
  - Phaepchromocytoma (adrenal gland tumor)
  - Skin cancer
  - Thyroid tumors
  - Prostate cancer
- Cannabis has been used to treat cancer for over 2,500 years; Ancient jars of cannabis have been found buried with their owners who were battling cancer.
- Certain strains of Indicas such as Purple Chemdawg (heavy body high, rest) and Hybrid's such as White Romulan (Pain relief, uplifting) prove to be most effective in helping cancer patients.
- A well-known Canadian named Rick Simpson used a strain called Romulan (indica) to create a cannabis hash/resin oil that he claims completely cured him of cancer. He educates thousands worldwide on this incredible medicinal plant. At Phoenixtears.ca you can read more about him and this amazing oil.

Health Tip 2
Reducing Inflammation

The cannabis plant contains hundreds of different substances that contribute to the anti-inflammatory components. Many people revere this plant. Cannabinoids are highly active compounds that help to inhibit inflammatory response. The effects of the external treatments can be felt in as little as a few minutes, while internally it may take up to an hour to feel the effects.

1. "Cannabis has long been accredited with anti-inflammatory properties." – Sciencedaily.com
2. Inflammation can be treated internally (capsules, tinctures, vaping, edibles) or externally with topicals (oils, creams and lotions).
3. Most of us have chronic inflammation (known as systemic inflammation) of some sort, add in the ingestion of daily toxins and that is what eventually leads to illness and life threatening diseases.
4. Reducing the effects of inflammation in your body will lead to a healthier lifestyle, suppression of pain, better sleep and less physiological stress.

Reducing Inflammation

- Some types of inflammation that may be treated with cannabis and hemp products:
  - Arthritis
  - Allergies
  - Sinusitis
  - Autoimmune disorders
  - Multiple Sclerosis
  - Colitis
  - Glaucoma
  - IBS and Crohn's
  - Strains/sprains
  - Joint swelling
  - Injury/surgery
- Many people use topicals, medicated bath salts or ingested cannabinoid treatments in order to find relief.
- In some states where cannabis is still illegal medically, hemp CBD treatments can be used for similar medicinal effects. Those types or remedies contain no THC and therefore will not give you any "high" effect.
- More and more health professionals are turning to holistic remedies to assist their patients in healing when modern medicine just won't do. The public is educating themselves to find earth-grown remedies and take their health in their own hands.

Health Tip 3
Alleviate Chronic or Acute Pain

More than 76 million Americans suffer from
chronic pain (pain that lasts over 6 months).
Using holistic remedies, including cannabis
products, to aid in suppressing chronic or even
acute pain (pain that lasts a few hours to a few
weeks) has shown to have astonishing results.

1. "...marijuana, helps people with chronic
   nerve pain due to injury or surgery feel
   less pain and sleep better..."
   Webmd.com.
2. Most people live day-to-day with some
   type of inflamed or irritated condition.
   They turn to self-medicating due to lack
   of insurance, funds, knowledge or time.
3. Using alternative, holistic products can
   be a - relatively - inexpensive way to
   help relieve some symptoms and break
   the pain cycle. Professional websites
   such as Earthclinic.com, Leafly.com,
   Planetearthremedies.com and
   All4naturalhealth.com (to name just a
   few) are all wonderful resources to
   educate yourself and find alternative
   choices for your personal health care
   needs.

Alleviate Chronic or Acute Pain

- The following are some of the chronic
  conditions and acute pain issues that different
  forms of cannabis therapies have shown to
  relieve.
    - Sinus pain
    - Back/neck pain & spasms
    - Arthritis/Joint pain
    - Tendonitis
    - Carpal tunnel syndrome
    - Fibromyalgia
    - Pinched nerve
    - Broken bones
    - Soft tissue damage
    - Menstrual pain
    - IBS and Crohn's Disease
- Cannabis has been used for thousands of
  years to treat the cramps, swelling and
  discomfort that come from PMS. Cannabis
  for premenstrual syndrome was used by
  Queen Victoria in the 1800s and its use dates
  back to Chinese women in 2700 BC.
- Cannabis has been shown to help with
  symptoms of chronic diseases like Irritable
  Bowel Syndrome and Crohn's Disease. It
  reduces swelling and stops nausea, diarrhea
  and abdominal pain.
- For years, cannabis products have been
  praised for the relief they have brought to
  painful conditions such as Rheumatoid
  Arthritis.

Health Tip 4
Soothing Various Skin Conditions/Injuries

There are many cannabis-infused topicals on the market today. "Cannabis-infused topicals are … known to have both analgesic and anti-inflammatory properties, making the plant perfect for use on surface-oriented pain." - Leafy.com/Aimee Warner of Cannabis Basics

1. Topicals help expedite the healing process for cuts, bruises, fractures and even wounds.
2. Hemp oil, which is used in many different topicals, has only trace amounts of THC, if any. It has no psychoactive properties and it is rich in omega fatty acids that our body needs for health. Hemp oil and seeds are abundant and can also be used in recipes when cooking.
3. "If you are a regular user of hemp oil products for the natural skin care, it acts as an anti-aging benefit too…it prevents skin disorders like psoriasis, eczema, acne and dry skin." – Seedguides.info
4. Creams, lotions, bath salts, oils and tinctures are all different kinds of products that can be used to alleviate a variety of mild to severe skin conditions or injuries.

Soothing Various Skin Conditions/Injuries

- Below are a few types of skin conditions and injuries where cannabis-infused products and other natural topicals have shown to be very effective in helping with relief in some way.
  - Psoriasis
  - Eczema
  - Bruises
  - After-surgery care
  - Dry, cracked skin
  - Wounds, cuts, scrapes
  - Softens scars, minimizes appearance
  - Red skin, rashes
  - Rosacea
  - Fractures and broken bones
  - Heals tattoos, stops itching
- "Eczema and psoriasis are conditions that are caused by atypical inflammatory response. Hemp seed oil has been shown to be effective in reducing symptoms of eczema and psoriasis…and Cannabinoids…have been demonstrated to have significant effect on chronic skin conditions." – Sensiseeds.com.
- Cannabis Basics, Kush Creams and Topical Way are all excellent, and proven suppliers of a variety of healing topicals and balms that you can find online.

Health Tip 5
Cannabis Helps Relieve Glaucoma

Glaucoma is a disease (eye condition) in which the optic nerve becomes damaged over time, reducing side vision within the eye. Glaucoma can cause partial, sometimes, total blindness. It affects over 60 million people worldwide.

1. The increased pressure and inflammation causes symptoms such as eye pain, blurred vision, reddening of the eye and halos around lights, among other things.
2. Treating glaucoma with cannabis has created some of the best documented studies available for using marijuana as a medicinal and remedial product.
3. There isn't a single valid study that exists that disproves marijuana's very powerful and popular effects with glaucoma patients.
4. Research studies have shown that smoking marijuana does lower eye pressure. Studies started as early as the 1970s showed that cannabis can be temporarily helpful with treating some of the symptoms of glaucoma.

Cannabis Helps Relieve Glaucoma

- The ways cannabis can relieve symptoms of glaucoma:
    - Reduces inflammation
    - Relieves eye pressure
    - Manages pain
    - Lowers blood pressure
    - Provides relaxation
- There are certain strains of cannabis that are more desirable to glaucoma patients for relieving pressure, pain and inflammation. Sativa strains such as Hawaiian sativa and Silver kush, along with Hybrid strains such as Sour power and Silver surfer have proven to be excellent for relief, according to glaucoma patients and research.
- "…recent research shows that marijuana may not only treat glaucoma by reducing eye pressure, but it may also act on certain receptors to provide a type of neuro-protection against damage to the optic nerve. This would treat glaucoma in a different way and is worth conducting further studies."
  – Vision.about.com

Health Tip 6
Treating Headaches and Migraines

Headaches are one of the most common disorders of the central nervous system. Migraines, which are severe recurring headaches, can last from 4 to 72 hours and are characterized by sharp pain and often accompanied by nausea, vomiting and visual disturbances. This type of debilitating pain can shut a person down for days at a time and affect all areas of their life.

1. "There are many reasons why people experience headaches, such [as] hormonal imbalances, food intolerances, liver intolerances, high or low blood pressure, structural misalignment, nutrient deficiencies, side-effects to medications, tiredness, stress or digestive complaints, and some headaches may be caused by simply being dehydrated." - Askanaturopath.com

2. Cannabis can be used effectively in treating pain and discomfort associated with headaches/migraines and dulls many of the symptoms. This allows someone affected to resume their normal day to day routine without the severe pain and other aliments associated with this disorder.

Treating Headaches and Migraines

- Some of the headache/migraine comfort that can be provided with ingesting, smoking or using cannabis creams include
  - Pain relief
  - Anti-inflammatory
  - Stress reduction
  - Provides relaxation
  - Dulls auditory/light sensitivity
  - Nausea
- Nearly 1 in 4 U.S. households include someone with migraines…many sufferers live in fear knowing that at any time an attack could disrupt their ability to work or go to school, care for their families or enjoy social activities. More than 90% of sufferers are unable to work or function normally during their migraine attacks. – Migraineresearchfoundation.org
- Hybrids such as Trainwreck and Indicas such as Sugar Mama are excellent strains for migraine and headache relief.
- "…marijuana was preventing the onset of migraines in vulnerable individuals. In addition, marijuana has long been known to possess analgesic properties." – PsychologyToday.com

Health Tip 7
Cannabis for Menopause Symptoms

Menopause is a change of human physiology that affects every single women when she passes her personal child bearing age (usually between ages 41-60). However there are many different levels and symptoms at which women experience it.

1. Indica-dominant strains are well known for the extremely effective pain relief they provide. For medicinal purposes and symptoms of menopause such as muscle spasms and insomnia, indicas usually are much more effective than sativas, although sativas can create an uplifting mood effect.

2. Depression, mood swings and hot flashes are the main complaints of women who are going through the menopause phase of their lives. Many women have claimed to have found relief when using cannabis treatments, from topicals on cramps to smoking or eating edibles for relaxation.

3. One woman claimed that smoking a small joint, barely enough to get the "high" feeling, alleviated her pain and hot flashes for 5-6 hours; after one or two "hits" off a joint, she stopped sweating immediately and the hot flashes subsided.

Cannabis for Menopause Symptoms

- Here are some of the menopause symptoms that can be relived with the use of cannabis treatments:
    - Mood Swings
    - Migraines
    - Back, joint and muscle pain
    - Depression
    - Stress and anxiety
    - Insomnia
    - Muscle spasms
- Qi Gong, acupuncture and herbal treatments are all excellent alternatives that can add balance to a regimen that includes cannabis.
- A hybrid such as OG Kush and an Indica such as God's Gift are recommended by women who have suffered menopause symptoms. Blue Dream is a sativa-dominant strain many women also like to use.
- "If you are going through or in menopause, at least consider marijuana as something which can improve the quality of your life… Cannadidiol (CBD) may also increase bone density, which is important as osteoporosis is a major concern for post-menopausal women." – Menopause-aid.blogspot.com

Health Tip 8
Cannabis and Dementia/Alzheimer's

Alzheimer's disease is a type of dementia that causes problems with memory, thinking and behavior. There are many stories and studies that show the benefits of using cannabis with someone who suffers from any type of dementia. One of the best results from using this medicine is the quality of life and contentment that seems to accompany using this natural remedy.

1. "Early studies suggest that marijuana may benefit weight gain and behavior in people who have dementia." – Mayoclinic.org

2. "Despite what you may have heard about marijuana's effects on the brain, the Scripps Institute, in 2006, proved that the THC found in marijuana works to prevent Alzheimer's by blocking the deposits in the brain that cause the disease." – Coed.com

3. Most dementia patients who use cannabis go from being angry, resentful and combative to friendly, calm and joyful. One of the reasons the tide is turning with the elderly, Alzheimer's and giving pot a try, is the extraordinary results that are being experienced.

Cannabis and Dementia/Alzheimer's

- A few of the main concerns that can improve when using cannabis as a treatment for different types of dementia include:
  - Helps behavior problems
  - Improves social skills
  - Increases motor skills
  - Slows brain degradation
  - Protects brain function
- "Gary Wenk, Ph.D, professor of neuroscience, immunology and medical genetics at OSU, told Time Magazine: "I've been trying to find a drug that will reduce brain inflammation and restore cognitive function in rats for over 25 years; cannabinoids are the first and only class of drugs that have ever been effective." – Naturalsociety.com
- "Researchers…recently published a cannabis study in the Journal of Neuroscience Research. …The study suggests that minuscule doses of THC [and cannabinoids] can prevent and heal cognitive deficits resulting from brain inflammation and other neurodegenerative diseases like Alzheimer's and Parkinson's." – Naturalsociety.com

Health Tip 9
Stop or Lessen the Frequency of Seizures

Epilepsy is a disorder that results from the surges in electrical signals inside the brain, causing recurring seizures. It is the 4th most common neurological problem. Over 2 million people suffer from epilepsy and even greater numbers experience some type of seizure. Many people are experiencing less frequent, or a cessation of seizures with the use of cannabis.

1. Seizures can be brought on by epilepsy or other issues in the body such as extremely low blood sugar, high fever, traumatic brain injury, brain tumor, withdrawing from drugs or a stroke.

2. According to the Mayo Clinic there are certain risk factors that increase your chance of having a seizure such as a family history of seizure disorders, sleep deprivation, medical problems that affect electrolyte balance, illicit drug use and heavy alcohol use.

3. "Early studies suggest that marijuana taken with antiseizure drugs may lower seizure risk in people with epilepsy... To treat epilepsy, 200-300 milligrams of CBD has been taken by mouth daily for up to 4.5 months." – Mayoclinic.org

Stop or Lessen the Frequency of Seizures

- Claimed benefits of using cannabis products as a treatment for seizures and epilepsy are:
  - Decreased seizure frequency
  - Relieves headaches
  - Less stress and anxiety
- Studies and patients who use pot to curb seizures seem to point to cannabis that is high in CBD (the major non-psychoactive ingredient in cannabis) and low in THC for the optimal results, which is to be seizure-free. These are strains such as Remedy, AC/DC, Harlequin, and Charlotte's Web.
- "The Epilepsy Foundation supports the rights of patients and families living with seizures and epilepsy to access physician-directed care, including medical marijuana. Nothing should stand in the way of patients gaining access to potentially life-saving treatment." - Epilepsy.com
- "Marijuana is a muscle relaxant and has "antispasmodic" qualities which have proven to be a very effective treatment of seizures. There are actually countless cases of people suffering from seizures that have only been able to function better through the use of marijuana." – Coed.com

Health Tip 10
Control Emotional Issues

The general population seems to think people only smoke pot to get high or treat a serious illness. There are many people that use it as a medicine to help control their emotions and depression, either daily or occasionally. There are even some mental disorders that are believed to be alleviated with cannabis use. Mood swings, anger, anxiety and stress are just a few emotions that can be managed, usually instantly relieved, with smoking or vaping cannabis.

1. "After years of feeling like a human guinea pig [switching] from one medicine to another... [a patient] decided to use medical marijuana to treat her depression and anxiety. [Although she is still] struggling with the same issues around love, neglect and abandonment—her moods, motivation and outlook are significantly improved by daily use of marijuana." PsychologyToday.com

2. Regarding ADD and ADHD "A well-documented USC study done about a year ago showed that marijuana is not only a perfect alternative for Ritalin, but treats the disorder without any of the negative side effects of the pharmaceutical." - Coed.com

Control Emotional Issues

- Cannabis has been known to help with mental and emotional issues such as:
  - Anxiety
  - ADD, ADHD
  - Depression
  - Not wanting to eat
  - Anger, Irritability
  - Insomnia
  - Bipolar Disorder
  - Lack of focus
- "In fact, cutting edge medicinal marijuana research suggests a joint a day might keep your psychiatrist away." – PsychologyToday.com
- "The European Neuropsychopharmacology journal has published a study that has confirmed the positive effect of THC to negative stimuli. The study, which was undertaken at the University Medical Center Utrecht in the Netherlands, claims that THC activates the endocannabinoid system naturally found in the brain to alter our response to negative images or emotions." - Dailymail.co.uk

Health Tip 11
Cannabis and Veterans, PTSD

Newly added to the list of aliments in WA state allowed for medical marijuana, along with traumatic brain injury (TBI), Post-traumatic Stress Disorder (PTSD) affects nearly 8 million American adults. PTSD becomes a personal disorder when someone experiences or witnesses a terrifying or dangerous event. The trauma memories can last months, years or a lifetime and affect more than just military veterans.

1. "The Food and Drug Administration has approved two types of antidepressants to help treat PTSD, but Hobbs said he thinks medical marijuana should be available as a treatment too." Thenewstribune.com said of Senator Steve Hobbs, WA state.

2. "...cannabis relieves symptoms of PTSD and anxiety so well that it has kept many veterans from committing suicide. "Without it, I wouldn't be alive today," said Randy Madden of Olympia, who said he suffers from flashbacks and anxiety stemming from his time in Iraq." – Thenewstribune.com

3. Women are twice as likely as men to get PTSD sometime during their life. It can affect anyone of any age.

4. High CBD strains are best for PTSD.

Cannabis and Veterans, PTSD

- Just a few of the ways that cannabis remedies can help PTSD and TBI sufferers:
  - Helps irritability
  - Assists with sleep
  - Lifts depression
  - Provides relaxation
  - Less self-destructive behavior
  - Calms nerves
- "If you have disturbing thoughts and feelings about a traumatic event for more than a month, if they're severe, or if you feel you're having trouble getting your life back under control, talk to your health care professional. Get treatment as soon as possible to help prevent PTSD symptoms from getting worse." – Mayoclinic.org
- "Research has suggested that cannabis may be a promising treatment option for a number of different physical and mental health conditions, from post-traumatic stress disorder to chronic pain." – Huffingtonpost.com
- Hybrid strains such as AC/DC, Harlequin, Remedy and Charlotte's Web are all excellent and effective high CBD strains.

Health Tip 12
Working with Cannabis and Eating Disorders

Anorexia is one eating disorder that is characterized by refusal to maintain a healthy body weight, intense fear of gaining weight and a distorted perception of body weight. Bulimia, binge/compulsive eating and obsessive dieting are also types of eating disorders.

1. "Most experts agree that eating disorders are characterized by a preoccupation with weight, body image, and/or food, but the reasons why an eating disorder develops are much more widely varied. An eating disorder can be an emotional, mental, or even a physical disorder."
– Symptomfind.com

2. "At least 24 million Americans have an eating disorder and these disorders have the highest mortality rate of any mental illness, according to statistics from the National Association of Anorexia Nervosa and Associated Disorders... about half of all people with eating disorders meet the criteria for depression...Research is finally paying attention to cannabis as a potential pharmacological medicine."
- Psyweb.com

Working with Cannabis and Eating Disorders

- Ways cannabis can help with eating disorders:
  - Create/encourage appetite
  - Alleviate depression
  - Help with anxiety
  - Emotional stability
  - Calming/relaxing effect
  - Break negative mental cycles
- "The ECS (endocannabinoid system) function and [Delta-9] THC have been found to aid in food consumption and appetite regulation along with many other bodily functions and behavioral reinforcements." – Psyweb.com
- "Physicians, psychiatrists and nutritionists are striving worldwide to show individuals with eating disorders that they are not alone and that help is available. The National Eating Disorders Association (NEDA) has information about health facilities, treatment options and diagnosis advice."
  - Symptomfind.com
- Eating disorders usually stem from past emotional, mental and family/relationship issues. It is important to talk to a professional for support, along with taking any medications, natural or otherwise.

Health Tip 13
Possible Alternative for Diabetes

Diabetes is a disease that affects over 170 million people worldwide with over 23 million in the United States alone. There are six deaths every minute due to complications of diabetes which equates to over 3 million deaths every year. The top 3 countries, in numbers of sufferers, are India, China, and the United States.

1. "Toking up may help marijuana users to stay slim and lower their risk of developing diabetes, according to the latest study, which suggests that cannabis compounds may help in controlling blood sugar." – CNN.com

2. "Three prior studies have shown that marijuana users are less likely to be obese, have a lower risk for diabetes and have lower body-mass-index measurements." – CNN.com

3. "Two other major actions of cannabis can benefit the diabetic. First is helping to keep blood vessels open and improving circulation. Cannabis is a vasodilator and works well to improve blood flow. Second, cannabis may reduce blood pressure over time."
   – Medicalmarijuana.com

Possible Alternative for Diabetes

- Ways Cannabis may be able to help control or eliminate diabetes:
  - ❋ Control blood sugar
  - ❋ Lower body-mass-index
  - ❋ Lessen need for insulin
  - ❋ Open blood vessels and improve circulation
- "Blocking the action of [cannabinoid] receptors may result in decreased motivation to eat, lower cholesterol and insulin levels, and increased glucose uptake…[THCV, a compound found in marijuana] may also help control excess liver fat, another sign of type 2 diabetes." – Healthline.com
- "Research published in the *American Journal of Medicine* has linked regular marijuana use to lower insulin levels, smaller waistlines and higher "good" cholesterol levels… Researchers… studied 4,657 [adults] from the National Health and Nutrition Examinations Survey (NHANES) between 2005 and 2010. Those who currently smoked marijuana exhibited lower levels of fasting insulin and lower levels of insulin resistance than those who never or occasionally smoked." – Medireview.com

Health Tip 14
MS, AIDS, and Spinal Conditions

There are many diseases and conditions which seem to be helped when someone uses cannabis as one of their chosen treatments. Today, many studies are being done to show the medicinal effects of this healing plant on many different ailments.

1. Marijuana has been studied for the relief of multiple sclerosis symptoms, such as nerve pain, muscle spasms, and urinary disorders. The active ingredients have an effect on the central nervous system and immune cells.

2. "Marijuana's effects on multiple sclerosis patients became better documented when former talk-show host, Montel Williams began to use pot to treat his MS. Marijuana works to stop the neurological effects and muscle spasms that come from the fatal disease." – Coed.com

3. "Benefits of Medical Marijuana in Spinal Cord Disease: THC has been shown to relieve symptoms and show significant beneficial effect on twitching, jerking and spasticity…It allows [the user] to experience minimal side effects and an increase in motor function." – Medicalmarijuana.ca

MS, AIDS, and Spinal Conditions

- Some of the symptoms that can be relieved by using cannabis:
    - Pain
    - Inflammation
    - Stiff joints
    - Nausea
    - Muscle twitching, spasms
- "THC and CBD's… bind to receptors in the brain and are effective against pain associated with conditions like multiple sclerosis and HIV/AIDS. By attaching to receptors, they block the transmission of pain signals." – Healthline.com
- "…The researchers injected mice that had an MS-like condition and partially paralyzed limbs, with CBD. The animals regained movement, "first twitching their tails and then beginning to walk without a limp." [They] noted that the mice treated with CBD had much less inflammation in the spinal cord than their untreated counterparts…they want to build on toward possible treatment for humans." – Medicalnewstoday.com
- "When used wisely, cannabis has huge potential…" Dr Kozela says."
    – Medicalnewstoday.com

Health Tip 15
Educating Yourself about Cannabis

With regard to the belief that states approving medical use will increase cannabis use in youth:

1. "The study administered by Dr Deborah Hasin, professor of epidemiology at Columbia University Medical Center is quite enlightening. The findings from 24 years of data from more than one million teens in the 50 states did not support the fears of increased adolescent use."
   – Coed.com

2. The organic cannabis plant is from the family of plants known as Canabaceae, which includes other plants like Hops and Hackberries.

3. "Marijuana (Cannabis sativa) has been grown in the United States since the early 1700s. Settlers brought the plant from Europe to produce hemp. Its use as a medicine was recorded in a reference book from 1850 titled "United States Pharmacopeia.""…

4. "According to a recent paper in The Journal of the International League Against Epilepsy, marijuana was used to treat a variety of conditions in ancient China as far back as 2,700 B.C."
   - Healthline.com

Educating Yourself about Cannabis

- Conditions treated by use of Marijuana in China, 2700 B.C. included: menstrual disorders, gout, Rheumatoid arthritis, malaria and constipation.
- There are still MANY people who are under attack for smoking or ingesting cannabis. So many old and improper stereotypes still linger in today's society. There are some who consider this a drug and not medicine. While it is agreed ANYTHING can be taken to excess; these people act in a very judgmental way toward those who choose cannabis as their personal, holistic remedy and use it in responsible ways. This is due to MANY years of propaganda, negative PR, miseducation, and improper studies.
- "I permitted my own years-long prejudices to move aside so that I can see more clearly what is right before my eyes. Science, not politics or prejudice, must be our guide. We must look with our own eyes without fear or prejudice. Only then can anyone expect to receive the best treatment possible."
  Dr. Jeremy Spiegel – PsychologyToday.com

You've finished. Before you go...

Tweet/share that you finished this book.
Please star rate this book.
Reviews are solid gold to writers. Please
take a few minutes to give us some itty
bitty feedback on this book.

ABOUT THE AUTHOR

Kat Bohnsack is a modern day gypsy and clairvoyant who teaches others about finding more effective ways to live their lives and grow closer to our source of power. She is also a speaker, educator, business owner, author, and a proud disabled veteran of the USAF. Kat comes from a family of active duty and disabled veterans across every war from Vietnam to Iraqi Freedom. She has dedicated herself to providing education, truth and answers to the decades long prohibition of a miraculous and organic plant that has a proven healing record spanning almost 5,000 years called cannabis.

Kat lives near Seattle, WA with her husband, Jeff, who is also a veteran committed to helping others. Kat works with the world's largest freedom of speech and cannabis event, Seattle Hempfest ®, she is an honored member of the prestigious group Women of Weed, featured in National Geographic, is considered an expert in her field and is associated with many businesses and groups who stand up for the rights of veterans, disabled persons and adults that choose this holistic herb (marijuana) for their personal health care needs. May freedom from persecution of any kind, reign and fill this world with peace, wisdom and kindness.

Other Amazing Itty Bitty™ Books

- **Your Amazing Itty Bitty™ Travel Planning Book** – Rosemary Workman
- **Your Amazing Itty Bitty™ Cruise Diary** – Itty Bitty Books
- **Your Amazing Itty Bitty™ Weight Loss Book** – Suzy Prudden and Joan-Meijer-Hirschland
- **Your Amazing Itty Bitty™ Food & Exercise Log** – Suzy Prudden and Joan Meijer-Hirschland
- **Your Amazing Itty Bitty™ Astrology Book** – Carol Pilkington
- **Your Amazing Itty Bitty™ Little Black Book of Sales** – Anthony Comacho
- **Your Amazing Itty Bitty™ Safety Book** – Stephen C. Carpenter, CSP
- **Your Amazing Itty Bitty™ Tax Audit Prevention Book** – Nellie Williams, EA

Coming Soon

- **Your Amazing Itty Bitty™ Business Tax Book** – Deborah A. Morgan, CPA
- **Your Amazing Itty Bitty ™ Book of QuickBooks® ShortCuts** – Barbara Starley, CPA
- **Your Amazing Itty Bitty ™ Heal Your Body Book** – Patricia Grarza Pinto